Lower his blood pressure in 14 days. 5 quick ideas for normal blood pressure and lowering hypertension. A guide to lowering hypertension naturally without medication.

By Thorsten Hawk

Content

The term blood pressure refers to the pressure of blood in a blood vessel. The decisive factor here is the force per unit area exerted between the blood and the walls of the vessels in the arteries, capillaries and veins. Blood pressure is mainly measured at the brachial artery (upper arm artery). In addition, it is vital because it can supply the organs of the human body with oxygen and nutrients.

The heart pumps blood into the main arteries and from there it is transported to the organs via a branched vascular system, so that the heart can supply the organs and tissue in the body with blood. With every heartbeat, the heart muscle contracts and blood is pumped into the large vessels of the bloodstream. This pumping process, which allows blood to flow, puts pressure on the elastic blood vessels. Thus, the pressure with which the heart pumps blood through the blood vessels of the organism is defined as blood pressure. In order for the blood to reach all organs and even the smallest capillary vessels, a certain pressure is needed to pump the blood out of the heart and to pass it on.

Since blood pressure is a dynamic quantity, hormone, vascular and nerve actions can influence it and it is normal and vital that blood pressure increases, for example in acute stress situations. Accordingly, the body reacts to demands in different situations and adjusts blood pressure accordingly.

Stress drives the heart to perform better, which in turn increases the blood supply to the muscles and improves their oxygen supply. In stressful situations, therefore, a higher pressure is needed to transport more blood to the stressed organs in the same time. The sympathetic nervous system, a part of the autonomic nervous system, is responsible for this. If necessary, this increases the power and frequency of the heartbeat, the small blood vessels constrict and the blood pressure can rise. On the other hand, the parasympathetic nervous system can cause the blood pressure to drop during resting phases. However, the level of blood pressure is also dependent on other factors. For example, the elasticity of the large vessel walls can have an influence on the pressure of the blood or the respective body position, as well as signals from certain hormones and nerves of the neurohormonal system. Furthermore, the resistance, which is determined by the vessel width, is also decisive. The greater the flow resistance, the more pressure is needed to push the blood through.

Blood pressure. What's normal?

During the course of the day, blood pressure is subject to natural fluctuations, which are perfectly normal in healthy people. The values are subject to a daily rhythm, the circadian rhythm, which is controlled by the autonomous nervous system. This means that blood pressure reaches its maximum value in the first two hours after waking up. Until early afternoon, the values drop slightly before rising again in the early evening hours. During the night, the blood pressure drops the most, so that the value can even be ten to 15% below the daytime value.

Blood pressure is measured in the unit "millimetres of mercury" (mmHg). The measured values are given in pairs. The World Health

Organization speaks of an optimal value when the upper value is below 120 and the lower value below 80 mmHg. Normal blood pressure is above these two values. However, as soon as the upper value rises above 140 mmHg and/or the lower value is above 90 mmHg, this indicates first-degree hypertension, i.e. high blood pressure. Two further classifications follow, second degree hypertension with an upper value of 160 and/or a lower value of 90 mmHg, and third degree hypertension with an upper value of 180 and/or a lower value of 120 mmHg.

Blood pressure measurement is simple, risk-free and necessary to obtain information about the cardiovascular system. However, reliable values can only be obtained if the blood pressure is measured for several days in a row and at rest. This means that you should wait about three minutes on a chair in a relaxed position before taking the measurement so that the circulation can come to rest. If the blood pressure is too high during several measurements or only one of the two values is elevated, this is known as high blood pressure.

Based on the first classification about the normality of the values, it is already apparent that blood pressure consists of two numbers. The higher upper value and the lower lower value. The first higher number stands for the heart value or the systolic value. This is the pressure measured during the heartbeat, i.e. when the heart muscle contracts to pump oxygen-rich blood into the circulation.

The lower number is called the vascular value or diastolic value. The pressure on the vessels is measured when the heart muscle relaxes. At the moment the muscle relaxes, the heart is filled with blood again.

Symptoms of high blood pressure

For more than 30 years, high blood pressure has been considered one of the most frequently diagnosed conditions in western industrialized countries and can therefore be described as a widespread disease. According to a comparative study, Germany is the country with the most high blood pressure problems in Europe. It is estimated that 20 to 30 million people are affected in this country. The age group or gender are irrelevant.

It is a clinical picture of the cardiovascular system in which the blood pressure of the vascular system is chronically elevated. The risk of hypertension rises with increasing age, so that in the over-55s nationwide, approximately one in two people suffer from high blood pressure. Nonetheless, young people can also be affected, as hypertension is favoured above all by overweight or lack of exercise. Initially, those affected show no symptoms whatsoever, so that high blood pressure is usually diagnosed late. The symptoms of the disease are also widespread, as there are no clear early symptoms. Usually the first signs only appear when the hypertension is very high. These symptoms include dizziness, headaches, which occur mainly in the early morning hours, sleep disturbances, nervousness, tiredness, or slight fatigue and shortness of breath. The face of the affected person is often reddened and secondary diseases can also indicate hypertension. These include, for example, water retention in the tissue, breast tightness or visual disturbances.

Why is high blood pressure dangerous?

High blood pressure is often described as a silent killer, because those affected sometimes do not even notice the disease or even feel particularly fit. Thus, the causes of health problems are only discovered in four out of five affected persons in the course of the illness, when serious consequential damage has already occurred.

Permanent high blood pressure has effects on numerous organs and bodily functions. Since the heart has to work harder if high blood pressure persists, the consequences are felt by the heart muscle. The muscles of the left ventricle become thicker and stronger, the walls thicken.

Muscle growth of the skeletal muscles is certainly desirable, but a thick heart muscle is not. The thicker the heart muscle is, the worse its oxygen supply is. In the long run, the heart becomes too weak to supply the body and its organs with sufficient blood and thus with nutrients and oxygen. As a result, this can lead to heart failure. At the same time, cardiac rhythm disturbances or sudden cardiac death due to thickened heart muscle can also be the result.

In addition, effects on the vascular system are possible. In principle, high blood pressure is a major risk factor for the development of arteriosclerosis. As a result of persistently high blood pressure, microscopically small injuries are formed on the inner wall of the vessels. This makes it easier for fats, proteins, cholesterol and also calcium to be deposited in the walls of the vessels. This leads to the formation of spot-shaped deposits, called arteriosclerotic plaque, which increase and calcify over time, resulting in the formation of arteriosclerosis. As a result, circulatory disorders of the underlying organs and muscles occur, as well as the formation of blood clots. Arteriosclerosis narrows the arterioles (small blood vessels) and this can result in cardiovascular diseases, such as a heart attack or cardiac insufficiency. Other consequences are coronary heart disease, strokes, arterial occlusive diseases and kidney failure.

Furthermore, elevated blood pressure can also have effects on the brain. About 15 percent of deaths among hypertensive patients can be attributed to strokes. There are several reasons for this. Increased pressure on the vessels in the brain increases the risk of a brain mass haemorrhage. In addition, arteriosclerotic constriction or blockage leads to a lack of blood supply to the brain if it is present in the brain itself or in vessels leading to it. This can take the form of a blood clot (embolus), for example.

The eyes can also suffer consequential damage if the blood pressure is permanently high because the blood vessels in the retina of the eye are very fine and chronic changes in the retinal vessels are caused. Suddenly occurring blood pressure crises, i.e. values above 210/110 mmHg, can lead to permanent damage to the retina with limitations of the field of vision and a decrease in visual acuity.

Damage to fine blood vessels in the kidneys is another problem of high blood pressure. Gradually the kidney loses its function, resulting in an estimated 10 to 15 percent of those affected experiencing kidney failure. Hypertensive nephropathy, i.e. a non-inflammatory disease of the kidney, which is accompanied by irreversible kidney damage, can also occur as a consequence of high blood pressure, since the increased protein excretion in the urine leads to impaired kidney function. In addition, constrictions or blockages are the reason for reduced blood flow, which reduces the kidney's capacity. Harmful substances can no longer be excreted sufficiently and the body tries to counteract this process. The kidney blood flow is increased with the help of the so-called RAAS (Renin-Angiotensin-Aldosterone System). However, this means that the vessels have to be narrowed and the blood pressure rises even more. This results in an eternal vicious circle.

Finally, effects on the aorta are also conceivable, since the aorta has to "absorb" the pressure with every heartbeat and pass it on (wind-chest effect). In the long term, the vascular walls are damaged and a vessel sacculation expands them in a sack-like manner. These aneurysms can then rupture and life-threatening bleeding can occur in the brain, chest and abdomen.

How to lower blood pressure quickly?

5 quick home remedies

Because of these consequences, an elevated blood pressure should definitely be lowered. Even a slight blood sedimentation of 5mmHg can prevent consequential damage. The risk of stroke is reduced by up to 15 percent and the risk of heart attack by up to nine percent.

Blood donations/Bleeding

Bloodletting or blood donation is a well-tolerated and at the same time drug-free treatment. Bloodletting is one of the oldest forms of medical treatment and alternative practitioners use this procedure to achieve a blood-lowering effect. It is a classic drainage procedure in which a certain amount of blood is taken from the patient. The aim is to rid the body of toxins and metabolic waste products and to stimulate blood formation and thus bring about a change in the organism. Nowadays, even a simple blood donation has an optional blood pressure-lowering effect.

A study of the citizens of Berlin Charité proves thereby that above all regular blood donation helps, in order to lower the blood pressure. A total of 292 patients participated in the study, 146 of whom suffered from high blood pressure with values of more than 140/90 mmHg. The remaining participants had normal blood values. Subjects suffering from high blood pressure were able to achieve an improvement in blood pressure values at the first blood donation. The participants who are not affected by the disease, however, did not feel any effects. Blood pressure remained within the normal range and hypotension, i.e. too low blood pressure can be ruled out as a result of the blood donation.

To ensure that the values could not be falsified, the test persons had to follow strict rules with regard to diet, sport or similar. In hypertensive patients it was found that the blood pressure continued to drop with each blood draw. On average up to 16 mmHg. Two advantages result from this test result. Firstly, it is a low side-effect and cost-effective therapy option for hypertension, and secondly, blood reserves are becoming increasingly scarce, so that the collection of blood is an advantage for seriously ill and emergency patients.

Sauna visit

Another way to lower blood pressure naturally is to visit the sauna, but this should be done with caution. In principle, a visit to the sauna is a good preventive measure. For example, a Finnish study shows that participants who visit the sauna four to seven times a week have a 45 percent lower risk of developing high blood pressure.

However, as a measure to reduce blood pressure, it is essential to consult a doctor beforehand to obtain information about the current condition. The body reacts to heat by warming the temperature of the skin surface, i.e. the outside temperature, by three to ten degrees Celsius. The core temperature inside the body increases by about one to two percent.

This process is therefore comparable to a fever and the body reacts in a similar way by activating the defence cells. The blood vessels expand and the heart rate is increased. As a result of the increased release of stress hormones of about 50 percent, the breathing rate increases and the muscles relax. About a quarter of a litre of sweat per quarter of an hour is produced in the sauna. The heat-induced dilatation of the blood vessels causes the blood pressure to drop. The German Society for Hypertension and Prevention describes the Sauna Effect as follows The upper systolic blood value rises with increasing length of stay in the sauna. The diastolic value rises at the beginning and then remains constantly elevated. Thus, there is no drop in diastolic values and the reduction in blood pressure only occurs during the resting phase, but then continues for a long time.

This means that those who have a well-adjusted blood pressure can use the sauna visit optimally to lower their blood pressure. In the long term, the sauna also has a positive effect, which is not only based on the aspect of sweating. Presumably, there is a functional improvement of the inner layer of arterial vessels, as well as a regulation in the release of stress hormones.

Nevertheless, some criteria should be considered. If a heart attack or stroke has recently occurred, the sauna should generally be avoided. The same applies to patients with recent blood pressure crises. If you feel dizzy, you should also leave the sauna immediately, as your blood pressure has probably dropped too much. In this case, a rest room should be sought to lie down. It is also worth mentioning and taking into account the fact that antihypertensive drugs have a stronger effect in combination with the sauna. The length of stay should generally only be three to five minutes at the beginning and then be slightly increased if well tolerated. In addition, after each visit to the sauna a rest break of at least 30 minutes should be taken and a jump into the cold water to cool down must be avoided at all costs. When cooling down, exactly the opposite happens, the blood vessels contract and this leads to a massive increase in blood pressure. It is better to take a hot shower and go for a walk in the fresh air afterwards.

Garlic has been considered for years as a home remedy to reduce high blood pressure, as it can prevent blood clots, which are usually caused by high blood pressure.

The food helps the blood clots dissolve in blood vessels and the spice prevents platelets in the blood from sticking together and causing blood clots. With the help of the two chemical substances contained in garlic, selenium and allicin, garlic has a preventive effect and lowers blood pressure, while at the same time automatically stopping the formation of blood clots.

In order for this effect to be successful, about one or two cloves of the garlic bulb should be taken every day. It is also possible to take garlic capsules, although this should also be taken daily. A study proves that daily intake of the capsules can reduce blood pressure by eight percent. Nevertheless, this household remedy is also associated with side effects that must be taken into account.

Particularly important are the interactions that arise from garlic consumption when taken in parallel with certain medicines. In addition, the breath and the smell of the skin will inevitably change and in rare cases gastrointestinal complaints can be caused. Care should also be taken when there is no hypertension, as daily consumption will still lead to blood sedimentation. This means there is a risk of having too low blood pressure in the end.

Camomile tea

Many health-promoting properties are also contained in chamomile tea and therefore it can also contribute to lowering blood pressure. There are three main reasons for this. The medicinal plant has anti-inflammatory and antispasmodic properties so that the vessels can relax and dilate.

This is important so that the blood can flow unhindered through the veins and arteries and a pressure build-up in the vessels is prevented. Camomile tea also helps to rid the body of excess salts and camomile has a calming effect. This can promote sleep and relieve anxiety and stress. Since a stressed and anxious state leads to an increase in blood pressure, these measures are particularly helpful if hypertension is associated with these aspects.

Dark chocolate

As a last household remedy, 90 per cent dark chocolate can be recommended, as certain ingredients of cocoa can lower blood pressure. 40 percent of the blood pressure reduction usually achieved by medication can be achieved with dark chocolate. However, caution is required when consuming it.

Too many calories can cancel out the positive effect on blood pressure. Likewise, normal chocolate is unhealthy for the heart, while dark chocolate with a high cocoa content and as little sugar as possible has a positive effect on the cardiovascular system. In general, the darker the chocolate, the healthier it is, because dark chocolate contains flavanols, vegetable substances that protect against arteriosclerosis.

However, these flavanols also ensure that the chocolate tastes bitter. For this reason, chocolate manufacturers usually remove the vegetable substances in advance and are not obliged to label the removal. In this way the beneficial effect of the chocolate is destroyed. For health benefits, an average of 53.5 milligrams of flavonoids should therefore be contained in each bar. A whole milk bar contains less than 14 milligrams and white chocolate contains no flavonoids at all. This means that "Dark Chocolate 90 Percent", which is particularly rich in cocoa and low in sugar, is the right choice if you want to feel a blood pressure-lowering effect.

High blood pressure Dietary basics

In order to understand the basic nutritional principles, it is first necessary to take a look at the causes of high blood pressure. In ten percent of all cases, organs or systemic diseases are the cause of high blood pressure. Then we talk about "secondary hypertension", which is usually caused by restricted kidney function or the narrowing of a renal artery. In this case, the treatment focuses on the underlying disease. In 90 percent of cases, however, "primary hypertension" is present, as no organic causes can be found. Certain factors additionally favour the occurrence of hypertension. For example overweight, excessive salt consumption, increased alcohol consumption, lack of exercise, nicotine or the influence of chronic stress. These factors should therefore be reduced as a preventive measure, but also as a treatment. The most important recommendations for a healthy lifestyle are therefore to aim for a normal weight, to consume little salt, and to maintain a moderate alcohol consumption. A balanced and appropriate diet, avoiding nicotine, regular physical activity, and a regular daily routine with breaks for rest and relaxation are also fundamental to achieve a lasting reduction in blood pressure.

In order to successfully reduce the intake of salt, canned food, ready-made meals, savoury pastries or salty fat dishes should be avoided, because salt is usually added to these foods during processing. Fresh and not already industrially processed foods, on the other hand, are low in sodium and have a positive effect on high blood pressure. The recommendation for a low-sodium diet is a maximum of six grams of table salt per day.

Foods that contain less than 120 milligrams of sodium per 100 grams include fruit, vegetables, potatoes, nuts or pulses, as well as tea, coffee, yogurt and quark. However, foods containing more than 400 milligrams of sodium per 100 grams should be avoided. These include smoked meat and fish products, sausage and cheese, ready meals, sauerkraut or potato chips.

Helpful nutritional tips are therefore to use common salt sparingly in the individual preparation of food and to use other spices and plenty of herbs. As a matter of principle, no more salt should be added at the table and fresh or frozen food should be preferred to canned food. In addition, mineral water should not contain more than 20 milligrams of sodium per liter. It is helpful to pay attention to the ingredients on the bottle and to information such as "suitable for low-sodium nutrition".

Alcohol intake must also be reduced so that blood pressure can be lowered. It is therefore advisable not to consume more than 20 grams per day, if possible.

On the other hand, a high potassium intake is beneficial, as potassium is the antagonist to sodium in the body and therefore weakens the effect of sodium on blood pressure. Potassium is particularly found in plant foods such as fruit or vegetables and potatoes. However, when cooking vegetables with lots of water, care should be taken to remove the potassium content, as the mineral is transferred to the cooking water and is thus lost.

Caffeinated coffee also increases blood pressure, but the blood pressure is only elevated for the next 20 to 30 minutes. For this reason, caffeine should not be consumed, for example through coffee, before measuring blood pressure. Overall, however, regular coffee consumption has a habituation effect, so that after two to three weeks the blood pressure increases are less pronounced or even no longer noticeable. Accordingly, coffee can also be consumed in a healthy amount in cases of high blood pressure.

In general, the diet should therefore be as low as possible in salt, sugar, white flour, red meat, smoked sausages, preserved foods, soft drinks and alcoholic beverages. However, fresh fruit, vegetables and herbs should be consumed several times a day, because if this diet is followed, normal weight can be achieved in the long term and blood pressure will drop. For every kilo less, about one to two mmHg can be deducted from the original values. Nevertheless, normal weight should not be achieved by drastic diets, as in the long term only a change in diet in combination with exercise is promising.

Foods that lower blood pressure

Especially unprocessed food oils with unsaturated fatty acids, such as rapeseed oil, are particularly effective in lowering blood pressure. Mineral water and unsweetened herbal and fruit teas are equally important antihypertensive agents. In addition, freshly cooked food should be used as often as possible and only herbs should be used instead of blood pressure-increasing table salt. Fruit and vegetables are also essential, as already mentioned, to achieve a reduction in blood pressure.

The best blood pressure reducers are folic acid, contained in cereal germs, yeasts, legumes or oranges, as well as omega 3 fatty acids, for example in herring, tuna or chia seeds. In addition, the ratio of omega 6 to omega 3 should be normalised, as a large part of the population consumes too much omega 6 but hardly any omega 3 fatty acids. The ratio of omega 3 to omega 6 should be between 1:3 and 1:5 if possible.

Potassium, which is found in bananas, nuts, spinach or tomatoes, and magnesium, which is found in wholemeal products or parsley, for example, also help to lower blood pressure. In general, a lot of vitamin D is also important for a healthy lifestyle. Therefore, at least 30 minutes should be spent daily in the open air in bright light.

Three whole grain products a day, such as oatmeal, have been shown to lower blood pressure by five to six mmHg. This is roughly equivalent to the effect of an antihypertensive drug and the risk of kidney or heart failure, stroke, aneurysms and heart attacks can be reduced by 15 to 25 percent.

Watermelons, for example, are particularly recommended fruit, as the amino acids they contain are converted to arginine in our body. This dilates the blood vessels and improves blood circulation. Watermelon thus counteracts a rise in blood pressure.

The potassium content in bananas is considerably high and this is beneficial for the fluid balance in our body and therefore also for the blood flow.

Kiwis are rich in antioxidants and for this reason, just like watermelons, they are rich in antioxidants, which helps the blood vessels and the blood can circulate better.

Most of the above-mentioned fruits are white-fleshed fruits that have a blood pressure-lowering effect, as they have a particularly positive effect on the heart. Nevertheless, an unbalanced diet should be avoided in any case.

Three large cups of hibiscus tea a day also help to lower blood pressure, as studies show. The blood pressure of the test persons should have decreased measurably within six weeks. The positive triggers are the anthocyanins it contains. These are responsible for strengthening the blood vessels and preventing them from contracting with increasing pressure. To prepare it, simply add two teaspoons of dried hibiscus flower to one litre of boiling water and leave to soak in for three to five minutes.

Many people also suffer from deficiency situations due to the choice of the wrong foods, so a doctor's opinion should always be sought when taking high-dose preparations such as magnesium or potassium. If in doubt, it is therefore healthier to consume foods with a particularly high magnesium or potassium content. A mismatch of potassium and magnesium adversely affects blood pressure and for this reason, a balanced diet should always be followed.

What kind of sport to lower blood pressure?

In addition to the right diet, sport also contributes significantly to lowering blood pressure. During physical activity, blood pressure initially rises, but in the subsequent resting phase, blood pressure drops. In order to avoid dizziness caused by a too high drop, there should always be enough fluid in the body. Accordingly, it is recommended to drink at least 1.5 to two litres of fluid. The amount of fluid you drink also depends on the outside temperature and the level of physical activity.

Sport can not only help to prevent high blood pressure in advance, because even a change from complete inactivity to light exercise is beneficial to health. With correctly dosed training, blood pressure can be reduced by five to ten mmHg, although this naturally varies from person to person, and the type of sport does not play a decisive role.

Endurance exercise is a good choice for the cardiovascular system. If the sports are not practised under competitive conditions and extreme ambition, jogging, Nordic walking, hiking, cycling, tennis or even swimming are ideal for lowering blood pressure. In addition, moderate strength training is recommended, as a larger muscle mass improves the metabolism and problematic insulin resistance can be reduced. This is present in many people with high blood pressure and a preliminary stage of diabetes. However, bodybuilding should not be done in a gym, as this training can lead to a dangerous overload of the cardiovascular system, especially in the beginning. In this respect, expert guidance is useful. This can also prevent incorrect breathing techniques.

Three to five training sessions a week are certainly appropriate, but in principle every movement is better than none at all. A unit should last about 30 minutes, but especially at the beginning a shorter duration of exercise can be useful. Especially if you haven't done any sport for years, you should start with a five minute training session and then slowly increase the amount of exercise. Instead of jogging, fast walking could be a good way to start, so as not to lose the fun of the sport. Overall, the intensity of the training should be noticeable, but the pulse rate should not increase too much. If you are uncertain, your doctor or cardiologist can also give you advice on how long you should exercise. In addition, the blood pressure should be checked before the sports programme and adjusted as well as possible to avoid serious consequences. Finally, the blood pressure rises sharply at first before it falls again.

Climbing stairs or giving up the car for the trip to the supermarket are suitable ideas for integrating sport into everyday life in general.

At the same time, yoga also has a blood pressure-lowering effect, relieves migraines and can stabilize patients after a heart attack. It is triggered by a combination of physical exertion, concentration and relaxation, as it stimulates the brain metabolism and produces more messenger substances that are important for the body's mental well-being. This includes, for example, the happiness hormone serotonin. Reversed postures, such as standing on your hands or head, should be avoided, as this increases the blood pressure in the head area, although it is precisely this effect that should be prevented.

All in all, sport can serve as a balance to the stressful everyday life and therefore relaxation, which is so often lacking nowadays, has a blood pressure-lowering effect. In addition, certain types of sport can lower the systolic value just as well as medication.

Legal notice:

I am not a doctor!

It is expressly pointed out that the tips, information, products and instructions presented here in no way replace a visit to the doctor.

This is not medical advice.

The information and texts presented here are not an invitation to self-diagnosis.

All texts and information are for informal purposes only. They have been carefully researched and checked, but no liability is accepted for the accuracy of all information.

Follow the tips at your own risk. Always consult your attending physician if you have health questions or complaints.

Imprint

© 2020 Randy Bolz

Sterndamm 17

12487 Berlin

Edition (1)

Cover design, Illustration: Randy Bolz

Editing, Proofreading: Randy Bolz

Translation: Randy Bolz

Publisher: Randy Bolz

Printers: Amazon Europe in Luxembourg